Ann Summers
SEXERCISE

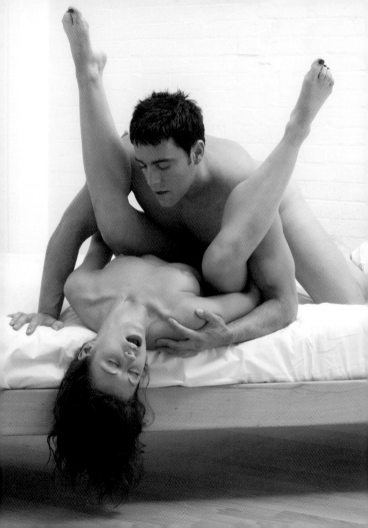

Ann Summers
SEXERCISE

EBURY
PRESS
LONDON

First published in Great Britain in 2006

1 3 5 7 9 10 8 6 4 2

Text written by Siobhan Kelly © Ebury Press 2006
Photographs © John Freeman 2006

First published by Ebury Publishing
Random House UK Ltd, Random House, Vauxhall Bridge Road,
London SW1V 2SA

Random House Australia (Pty) Limited
20 Alfred Street, Milsons Point, Sydney, New South Wales 2061, Australia

Random House New Zealand Limited
18 Poland Road, Glenfield, Auckland 10, New Zealand

Random House South Africa (Pty) Limited
Isle of Houghton, Corner Boundary Road & Carse O'Gowrie,
P.O. Box 2002, Houghton 2041, South Africa

Random House UK Limited Reg. No. 954009
www.randomhouse.co.uk

A CIP catalogue record for this book is available from the British Library

Art direction and design by Smith & Gilmour, London
Photography by John Freeman

ISBN 0091909252

Papers used by Ebury are natural, recyclable products made from wood
grown in sustainable forests.

Printed and bound by Tien Wah Press

Designed and typeset by Smith & Gilmour, London

Contents

Foreword 7

Introduction 8

Exercises 14

Genital Exercises 29

Warm-up 34

Food of Love 42

Positions 55

Mind, Body, Spirit 79

Cooling Down 90

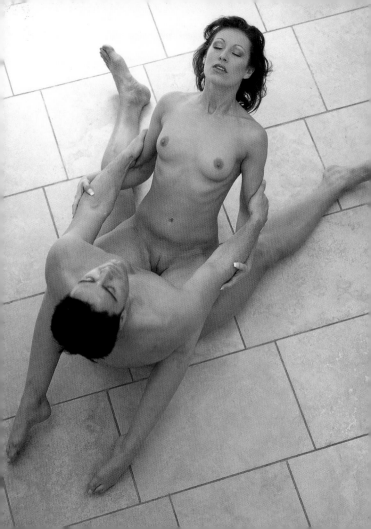

Welcome to Ann Summers SEXERCISE.
Our LITTLE BOOK OF SEX and RED HOT &
RUDE POSITIONS have already inspired
lovers everywhere to spice up their sex
lives – now SEXERCISE will help you get
fit while you´re having fun! A healthy
body makes for good sex and a healthy
relationship, and you don´t even need to
go to the gym every day: a steamy bedroom
workout can burn off as many calories as
a session on the treadmill. Boost your heart
rate and get your blood pumping, and you
will not only increase your pleasure but
keep going for longer! Don´t be afraid to
get a bit of Sexercise in your life.

Enjoy!

Jacqueline Gold,
CHIEF EXECUTIVE ANN SUMMERS

LET'S GET PHYSICAL!

Welcome to **Sexercise**, a brand new concept combining orgasmic sex moves with workouts and food to get your body bed-hot.

Good health and good sex go together. Not only do fit, healthy bodies promote self-esteem and physical health, toned and flexible muscles will enable you to make love in those acrobatic positions you've always longed to try but thought were only possible for Olympic athletes and circus contortionists.

The truth is, Sexercise is open to everyone, whatever your current level of fitness: a little light exercise, a nutritious aphrodisiac-packed diet and a spirit of adventure in the bedroom could open the door to the sex life you've always wanted. It's easy to think of exercise as gruelling, but making love is a fabulous – and free – way to keep fit in itself. Sex is a great mood-booster and a fun calorie-burner, too: energetic sex burns about seven calories over five minutes – so keep it up for two hours, and you'll burn 168 calories.

Fitness just got a whole lot sexier . . .

HEY, GOOD-LOOKING!

While the world would be a dull, dull place if we all had identikit muscle-man or Barbie-doll bodies, it's undeniable that people who move around more look – and feel – better in their own skin. Exercise has been shown to promote body image. Women and men surveyed after attending the gym reported finding their body sexier on the way out than on the way in.

And, in turn, a healthy body image increases **desire**, especially for women. It doesn't take a genius to work out that the woman who's comfortable in her own skin is more likely to make love with the lights on, experiment with new positions and revel in the attention her lover pays her. There's nothing sexier than a woman who's confident in her own sensuality.

There have been dozens of surveys conducted to research the effects of regular exercise on sexual desire and performance. The happy, horny news is that pretty much all of them reach the conclusion that active people get more and better sex than couch potatoes.

Exercise gets blood pumping round the whole body – genitals included. And blood circulation is key for a man's erection (it's increased blood flow that makes his member stand to attention) and a woman's arousal system (more blood to the genitals increases lubrication and clitoral swelling). Your flushed cheeks and glowing skin show the benefits immediately – in fact, the physiological changes that your body undergoes after a good workout and great lovemaking are very similar, meaning that when we see someone sweaty and fresh from the gym our brains make the subconscious connection between arousal from the gym and sexual arousal. When you exercise, heart rate and blood pressure are elevated and the blood vessels in the genitals become primed for action.

FACT: HEALTHY BODIES HAVE BETTER SEX

After a good workout, your body releases **endorphins** into the bloodstream: these hormones act as natural painkillers, so if you're active, you'll never need to cry off sex because you've got a headache.

One survey found that **regular sex** helps you look between four and seven years younger because it helps you feel more content, sleep better and feel less stressed. **Orgasm** helps you sleep which is also important for your immune system, your stress levels, your performance at work and your libido. Exercise stimulates the endocrine glands, which make testosterone levels in both men and women rise sharply. And high testosterone levels mean high levels of sexual desire and performance. It also boosts oestrogen levels in women, which makes the skin look younger, firmer and healthier.

In fact, exercise is such a powerful **sex-booster** that research from the University of Texas at Austin suggests that women who have problems with sex drive, arousal or orgasm should do something arousing like working out to get stimulated. Who needs Viagra when a brisk walk in the woods will do the trick?

Exercise keeps nerves in tip-top shape, sharpening the ability to feel and focus on all bodily sensations.

Men on the move can have sex more frequently: after a few months of working out for one hour, three times a week, a man is likely to have a shorter post-ejaculation recovery period. His increased cardiovascular fitness (that's stronger heart and lungs) will also mean that he's got extra stamina for Round Two. *Ding ding!*

FACT: SEXY BODIES HAVE BETTER HEALTH

Men who get horizontal three times a week cut their risk of a heart attack in half.

People who have sex twice a week live longer because sex helps to raise the substances that lengthen life span, dehydroepiandrosterone (DHEA), oxytocin and endorphins – and lower those that can shorten it – cortisol and adrenaline.

Those who exercise regularly have more sex and experience better and more satisfying orgasms than those who live more sedentary lives. Women get **aroused** more quickly and men achieve **stronger erections**.

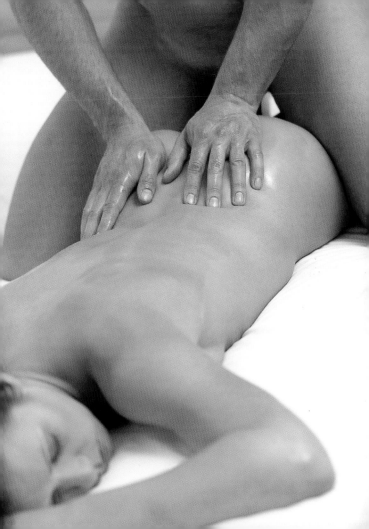

SEXUAL FITNESS: YOUR ESSENTIAL KIT

Healthy sex is **safe sex**, and responsible lovers equip themselves with basic equipment and health and hygiene rules:

- It's worth visiting a **sex clinic** to have your system checked for sex bugs before you even think about having unprotected sex within a committed relationship.
- Sharing **sex toys** is a bad idea because body fluids and bacteria can hide in every nook and cranny: clean them out with warm soapy water, freshen them up with special alcohol cleaning wipes or slip condoms over them before you use them to be 100 per cent safe.
- **Oral sex** carries a risk. Unless you and your partner both have a clean bill of sexual health, use a dental dam for either oral sex or rimming (using a tongue to stimulate a partner's anus), and don't swallow your partner's semen.
- Remember that **STIs** can be caught via any genital contact, not just ejaculation.
- **Condoms** are the safest way to protect your body from STIs. Check out the right kind of condom for you: polyurethane condoms are available for those who don't like latex or are allergic to it. Make sure they bear the British Standard mark which means they've been tested and provide good protection against STIs and pregnancy. Check the expiry date and don't use old damaged condoms that have been open for a while.
- **Anal sex** is a particularly high risk without a condom so choose one designed to cope with the rough-and-tumble nature of backdoor loving. It's also vital that you use a lubricant: the anus doesn't produce its own natural juices when aroused, so flesh can tear and become vulnerable to infection.

MOTION LOTION:
THE IMPORTANCE OF LUBRICANT

Even the healthiest bodies sometimes need a little extra help during sex. While women make natural sex juices when they're pumped up and ready to go, there are various reasons why she might not get as wet as she needs to for sex to be comfortable.

Water-based lubricants, like **KY jelly**, are by far the most commonly used and are great for play and penetration. They are safe to use with condoms and are often slightly sweet because of their glycerine content, so can be used in oral sex. However, they can dry out quickly, which means during a marathon lovemaking session you'll need the tube to hand.

Silicone-based lubricants are the clever new kid on the block: they're completely waterproof and don't dry out. You only need a tiny amount, but the downside is that you need soap and warm water to get rid of all traces. They're compatible with most condoms but can erode silicone sex toys.

Petroleum-based lubes like **baby oil** or **Vaseline** are often used because we happen to have them in the home. But they're not designed to enter our bodies, so are better for male masturbation. They will also dissolve condoms if the oil touches the latex – you have been warned!

Purpose-made **oil-based lubricants**, available from some sex shops, are good for dildos and anal penetration but again, are incompatible with condoms. They also stain easily, so avoid them if you don't want your bedsheets to tell visitors exactly what you've been up to (and where on the bed you got up to it).

Food-based or **flavoured lubricants** are also popular. If you or your partner is susceptible to thrush, avoid anything containing sugar or glycerine as food-based lubes are notorious for triggering yeast infections.

EXERCISES

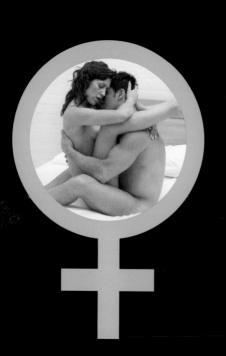

MOVES TO SHAPE YOU UP

Trying the sex moves in this book could be the best thing you ever do for your love life, but some of the positions that are designed to give you a workout are best attempted by fit, healthy bodies: you'll never reach orgasm if you have to stop for a breather every two minutes, or your leg muscles can't bear your partner's weight, or you're not flexible enough to wrap your limbs around your lover's neck.

So to get the best out of sex you're going to have to lose the flab, tone that body and get healthy. But you don't need to set up camp in the gym or become a yogic guru to achieve this. Doing serious exercise (the kind that leaves you out of breath) for half an hour, three times a week is all it takes. You'll see the results in your wellbeing and your looks within a fortnight. Working out too much means your muscles will be sore, you'll be fatigued and if you're too tired and sore to leap into bed, the hottest body in the world is no good to you.

If you can get to a gym, try aerobic exercise – a workout that leaves you out of breath, but able to have a conversation – with some light weight training and a healthy diet. If you can't get to a gym, the good news is you can exercise anywhere, from your living room to your local pool or a nightclub – so no excuses!

Running a mile three times a week will shape up your legs, burn fat and boost your performance in the sack. Two-thirds of runners said regular jogging made them better lovers. Cycling will also tone your lower body and is excellent for overall fitness, and what's more, 66 per cent of biking enthusiasts said cycling improved their sexual performance. Making a splash will keep you horny well into middle age and beyond: swimmers over 40 were as sexually active as those in their twenties. Pilates makes your body appear longer and

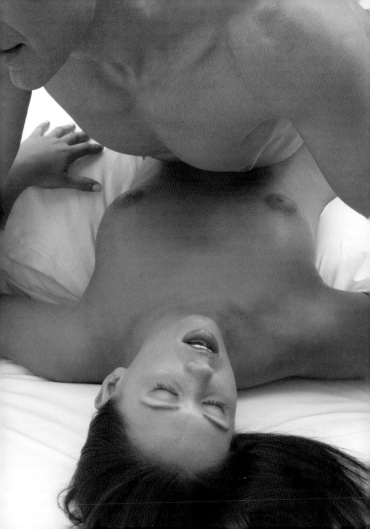

leaner, and is unbeatable for honing your PC muscles
(see pages 30–33). Yoga increases your body's flexibility,
making it easier for you to assume positions that involve
wearing your ankles as earrings. A salsa class with your
partner will not only give you a great aerobic workout but is
also a fun, intimate, unusual way to spend an evening together.

And it's not just about sculpting your arms or reducing
your waistline. Increased cardiovascular output during
exercise raises the amount of adrenaline in the body, meaning
you're ready for an adventure. Directly after vigorous exercise,
you're more likely to experiment with demanding, daring
positions that will take your sex life to new heights.

Increased blood flow throughout the body increases arousal,
sensation, lubrication and the intensity of orgasm during sex.
Plus, exercise releases a huge surge of endorphins, a.k.a. the
'happy hormone', into your bloodstream. Endorphins are nature's
painkillers and stress relievers, so all the day's worries, aches
and pains take a back seat while you concentrate on ravishing
each other. So forget traditional dates like the cinema or posh
restaurants: exercising with your partner is the best way to
ensure you're both primed for intense, vigorous, acrobatic sex!

GET A HOT BODY, ZONE BY ZONE

We've all got a favourite erogenous zone – that part of the
body that melts under your lover's caress. Whatever yours is,
it's going to be receiving a lot of attention in the near future –
so hone and tone it with these specific body-sculpting moves.
To get the most out of these exercises, combine them with
aerobic activity – a twenty-minute jog or brisk walk beforehand
should be enough. It's important your muscles are warmed
up and flexible before you attempt these exercises.

Bum

Anyone who grew up riding horses will tell you that staying in the saddle gives you a high, toned butt to die for. But horseriding is not always the most practical way to work out, especially if your gym has a no-horse policy. The good news is the glutes – the muscles in your bottom – are the largest muscles in the body and exercises to tone them up are simple, if not exactly easy. Try butt kicks. Kneel on all fours, extend your leg behind you and raise it up, then repeat. For a variation on the theme, try tiny, fast up and down movements.

If you like this move, you'll love this position: Wheelbarrow, page 67, shows off a toned, round butt.

Arms

Rowing is a great way to define your whole upper body, or if you'd rather work out at home, try this move. Tricep dips work on the triceps, the muscles along the back of your arms that can turn into 'bingo wings' if they become flabby. Sit on the side of a chair or bench. Place your hands on the edge of the chair, right on either side of your butt, and grip. Move your body forwards, keeping your hands firmly on the chair. Now dip your whole body down, bending your arms. Go down as far as you can and then slowly raise your body back up: you'll feel the burn as your triceps are squeezed. If you've never worked out this muscle group before, it's fine if you can only manage one or two squeezes: aim to work up to three sets of twenty tricep dips for arms that any lover would want to be wrapped in.

If you like this move, you'll love this position: 69, Woman on Top, page 71, requires every bit of the strength you've built up in your arms!

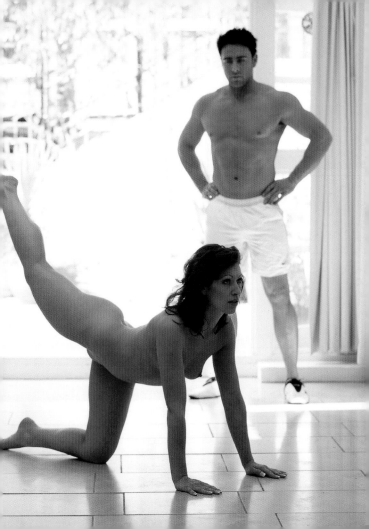

Bust

Swimming is excellent for improving the muscles that support your bust, but these standing push-ups work just as well at toning your entire pectoral area. Stand facing a wall with your feet about 60 cms (two feet) from the skirting board. Place your hands on the wall, shoulder-width apart. Bending only at the elbows and keeping your body stiff and straight, lower yourself forward towards the wall then push yourself away from it.

If you like this move, you'll love this position: The Crunch, page 76, means you're both eye-level with each other's chest.

Legs

Hitting the ice rink or strapping on your rollerblades strengthens your inner thighs (a typically weak area for women), which can make intercourse more exciting. Tone these muscles and you'll find that when you squeeze them together during sex, the walls of your vagina feel tighter. Do plié squats. Put your hands on your hips, place your feet more than shoulder-width apart and turn your toes out slightly. With your torso upright, squat until your hips are almost parallel to your knees. Hold for two counts then return to the starting position. Try to work up to two sets of twenty squats.

If you like this move, you'll love this position: Thigh Mistress, page 58, was designed to show off strong, toned thighs.

Tummy

When you do sit-ups, your pelvic muscles, which contract during orgasm, also get a workout. And the stronger those muscles are, the more intense your climax will be. To engage your pelvic muscles while you do your sit-ups, make sure your lower back stays on the floor and keep your shoulder blades

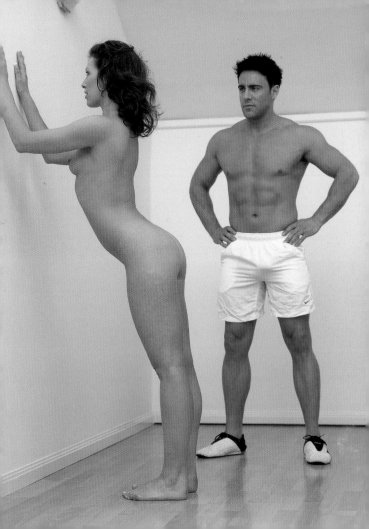

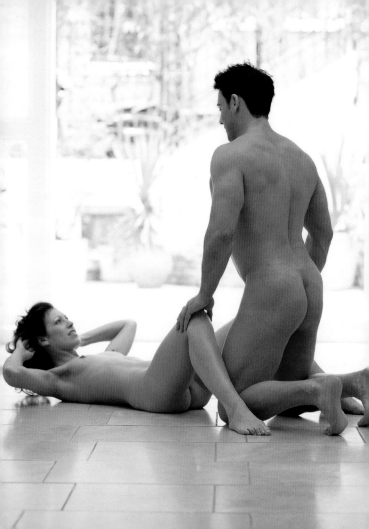

lifted up off the ground the entire time. Do three sets of fifteen crunches three times a week and within two weeks, you'll notice that not only are your abs stronger and your stomach flatter but your pelvic floor is stronger too.

If you like this move, you'll love this position: The Mexican Wave, page 73, shows off a flat tummy and needs strong abdominal muscles.

STRETCHES FOR TWO

Stretches are one of the most important parts of any exercise regime. Cardiovascular work is essential for fitness and weight-bearing work builds strength, but if your muscles aren't loose and relaxed, then you won't be able to relax and experiment in bed. Tight, short muscles limit the range of motion of the legs, hips and pelvis, all key players in sexual activity. In addition most of us clench our muscles. Stretching pumps a lot of blood into muscles and that stimulates the nerves that run through them.

Done every time you exercise these stretches will keep you limber, flexible and ready for some bedroom acrobatics at a moment's notice. Some of these stretches might take you beyond your current range of movement. You should feel tension but never pain: breathing slowly and concentrating on every breath can help you get through a tough stretch.

Imagine a demanding sex position you've always wanted to try but never dared. Do it fully clothed as stretches: instead of bumping and grinding, just hold the position, using each other to balance and supporting wobbly arms and legs where necessary. This works on two levels. Firstly, this dress rehearsal gets you both excited about the actual performance. Secondly, you don't risk injury by attempting something that's a little beyond your range in the heat of the moment.

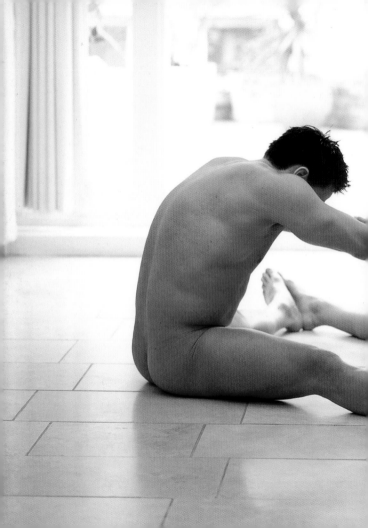

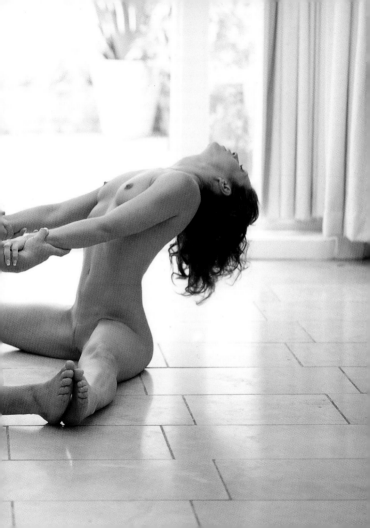

Sit facing your partner with your legs wide apart and the soles of your feet touching his. Draw your feet towards your pelvis and gently press the soles together to increase the stretch. Hold for one to two minutes until your muscles are completely relaxed into the stretch, and look into each other's eyes.

Remain sitting with the soles of your feet touching and stretch a different muscle group: keeping your backs straight and tall, spread your legs in a wide V shape until you can grab each other's hands. Lean back as far as you can, pulling him gently forward, and feel the stretch in your inner thighs. Then lean forward while he leans back and feel your glutes lengthen and relax.

Kneel on your feet. Lean forward, resting your torso on the top of your thighs, arms forward so that your spine is elongated and stretched. Your partner stands directly behind you and gently presses your back to push you beyond your comfort zone. Switch places and repeat: the benefits of having a looser, freer spine manifest themselves in almost every sexual position.

Sit with your legs apart, his feet above your ankles. As you relax forward he gently pulls your arms to deepen the stretch. Repeat daily until you're flexible enough to plant a kiss on his lap or administer oral sex from this position.

The hamstrings, or backs of the thighs, often suffer if you sit down at work all day – but need to be limber for adventurous sex. Put your foot up on a bench or raised surface that you are standing in front of. Use your partner to balance. Lean over and try to touch or grab your foot. For the greatest stretch, keep your lower back arched as you lean over.

WORKING UP A SWEAT: NATURE'S LOVE POTION

Don't be in such a hurry to jump into the shower after your workout. The scent of fresh perspiration is actually an aphrodisiac. Natural body odour has been regarded as the most potent of sexual scents throughout human history. Even though the French produce much of the world's most famous perfumes, they also find the body's natural scent sexual and call it *la cassolette*, slang for 'perfume box'. In Shakespeare's time, a woman hoping to attract a man tucked a peeled apple in her armpit and then offered this love apple to the object of her lust. So why should you pounce on your lover fresh from the gym? Well, perspiration is packed with subtle, complex scents called pheromones. This come-hither aroma is a sexual signalling mechanism to let males know when females are ready to mate.

Pheromones have a slow, subtle effect and work after prolonged exposure (so it's a gradual process of arousal rather than the 'one sniff and she will be mine' of the mythical Love Potion Number Nine). Scientists have discovered a chemical pheromone that men exude from the apocrine glands in the armpits and genital area. A study has shown that women either smell or absorb this pheromone in men's natural body odour during intimate sexual contact, and that it makes women sexually aroused and even healthier. The study showed that women who have sex with a man at least once a week have regular menstrual cycles, milder menopause and are more fertile, compared to women who are celibate or having irregular sex. Women possess pheromones too. In fact, unlike the male essence, which requires direct contact to have an impact, the female essence can disperse across a room.

Research indicates that this aromatic female pheromone works on other women as well as men. Scientists are working on bottling this magical aroma, but as yet, there's no product as powerful as nestling into your lover's arms.

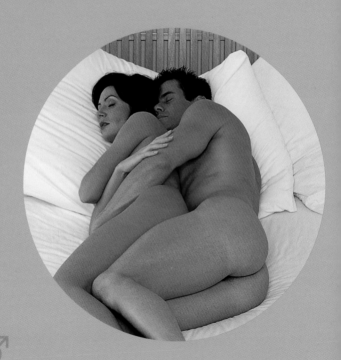

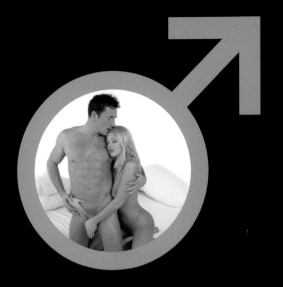

GENITAL
EXERCISES

PUMP UP YOUR LOVE MUSCLES

Everyone knows about working the muscles that make us look good – but keeping your internal muscles in tip-top condition is essential for Olympic-standard sex. If any muscle doesn't get used, it loses its strength and the muscles around the genitals are no different. The good news is, exercising your sex muscles is easy, you can do it in secret, you won't break a sweat – and you'll feel the benefits instantly.

The delicious sensation you get when you reach orgasm is essentially a contraction of your pelvic floor muscles, which reach from your anus to your pubic bone and stretch all the way round your abdomen. The medical name for this magic ring of muscle is the pubococcygeus muscle, or **PC muscle** for short. It doesn't take a sports science degree or a diploma in sexology to work out that the stronger this muscle is, the stronger your contractions will be, and the more control you will have over your and your partner's sexual satisfaction.

The power of the PC muscle is a relatively recent discovery. In 1952, Dr Arnold Kegel was conducting research to help incontinent people achieve better bladder control, and hit on the method of stopping and starting the stream of urine mid-flow. And a wonderful accidental discovery was made: his female patients not only learned to control their waterworks but also found their sex lives improved almost overnight. Their stronger vaginal muscles meant that sensations during intercourse were radically amplified – and the orgasms, when they came, were bedrocking. Their husbands weren't complaining either as the muscles became snugger, hugging the penis even tighter during sex.

And it's not just women who benefit: many men say stronger PC contractions stimulate the prostate gland, which passes

through the muscle, and is aroused when he ejaculates.
It also helps him to control when he ejaculates, and can make
his erection last longer.

THE WILLY WORKOUT: PC EXERCISES FOR HIM

The PC is an important muscle, but many men don't know
where it is or how to locate it. The prostate gland and the
urethra pass through the PC muscle, which runs from the
tailbone up to where the penis attaches to the pubic bone.
Because it connects the front, the back and all the bits inside,
it stands to reason that if you strengthen the PC muscle, you
can increase control and sensation in the entire genital area.

The best way to locate your PC is to stop and start the
flow when you're peeing: you should feel the muscle contract.
Feels quite nice, doesn't it? A word of warning: restarting
the flow can be messy, and it takes a bit of practice, but once
you've mastered the art of stopping and starting you're ready
to move on to the next phase of your PC workout. Once a day
is plenty of practice: any more and you risk giving yourself
a kidney infection.

To take it to the next level, lie back on your bed and relax
the muscles in your thighs, bottom and abs. Now tighten
and draw in your anus as though you were trying not to fart,
and hold your urethra as if you're trying not to urinate. It
should feel as if you're lifting them up and squeezing them
from inside. Hold the contraction for three seconds and then
slowly release. Repeat it as many times as you can: over the
course of a week, add one more contraction each time until
you can comfortably manage twenty contractions. Once you're
really comfortable, you can even do this at your desk at work.
Sorry boys, but strengthening the muscle won't bulk it up . . .

Advanced workout

Once you've mastered control of your PC muscles, you should find you're able to control when you climax during sex. If you want to gain even greater command over your erection, put a piece of kitchen roll over your erection and see if your penis can hold the weight. Graduate to a face cloth if you can manage it, but never hang weights off your penis, despite what you've seen martial artists do on holiday – your penis can break, and this is one sports injury that's really not worth the risk.

MUSCLE MANIA: PC EXERCISES FOR HER

The PC muscle is located about 2 cm (1 inch) inside the vagina and runs from the tailbone at the back to the pubic bone in the front. To locate it, sit on the toilet, spread your legs and stop and start the flow when you're peeing. The muscular sensation you feel is your PC muscle working (as with men, do this sparingly and only until you're sure you've found the muscle – constant stopping and starting can give you a bladder infection).

When you've found your PC muscle, lie back on your bed and contract it. Put a finger in your vagina and squeeze and you'll feel it working. Try to focus on your vaginal muscles: your back and buttocks will involuntarily clench, but keep them as relaxed as you can. When you've got the hang of this incredibly easy exercise, you can practice your PC squeezes anywhere. Some women even reckon they can bring themselves to climax just by doing it, so beware of powerful public orgasms!

Gradually build up to twenty contractions a day, varying long squeezes with lots of short, sharp clenches. Do six sessions a day and you'll soon have strong, healthy PC muscles.

Advanced workout

Put a slim vibrator or dildo inside your vagina and see if you can move it in and out just using your PC muscles. Once you've mastered that, treat yourself to a vaginal barbell or love balls, which you insert into your vagina, then use your PC muscles to hold them in place – it's an incredibly sexy secret.

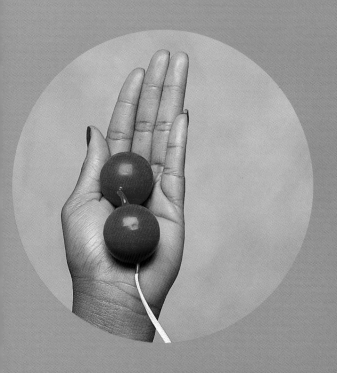

WARM-UP

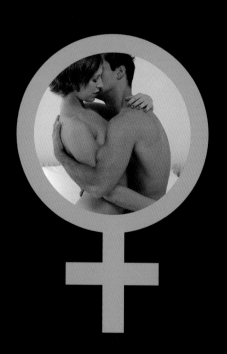

THE WARM-UP: WHY FOREPLAY PAYS

Just as you have to warm up before a workout, you can't expect to have great sex without **foreplay** – the stroking, kissing, caressing and talking that builds up to the act of penetration. Sure, sometimes a sexual sprint – a quickie session that's over in three minutes – is just what you want, but more often than not, foreplay is the key to great orgasms. These warm-up tips can be used before intercourse in your favourite position or as everyday bonding rituals.

The pre-sex ritual of kissing and caressing is a pastime in its own right. To really win her over, he should do lots of it even when he doesn't want penetrative sex. That way, her body will be constantly primed and ready for sex: you're building up a knot of tension you'll finally release with orgasm.

Never underestimate the power of **kissing**: ancient sex gurus believed the lower lip was connected directly to the clitoris, and current sexologists acknowledge that many women become aroused and lubricated after a good snog – some women lubricate more through passionate kissing than they do through genital stimulation. Kissing each other on a daily basis for pleasure rather than as a preamble to sex will ensure your bodies are always slightly stimulated and primed for acrobatic lovemaking at a moment's notice.

It can be tempting to go straight for each other's genitals but linger over other parts of the body first. Experiment with light tickles and stronger, definite strokes: use props from fluffy feathers to spanking paddles depending on the intensity of touch your partner desires. And most importantly, keep talking to each other, giving positive feedback when your partner's turning you on, and gently but firmly telling them when a particular move doesn't really work for you.

Try **bodymapping**: identify and memorise your lover's erogenous zones and you've got a sex slave for life. Ask him to caress you and rate his touches on a scale of one to ten for each body part. This is the best way to find out and remember where you're most sensitive. So, your inner thighs might score a touch-me-there ten, while your arms are less sensitive and only rate three. Then return the favour, making a mental note of the places he loves to be touched. Everyone has different erogenous zones, so do this with every new lover.

She can trail her breasts all over his body. The friction of his skin underneath her nipples will stimulate her, and the sight and texture of her breasts giving his skin a light massage will have him begging for more.

There's a discrepancy between men and women when it comes to foreplay: men can be ready for penetration in a matter of minutes while women take an average of twenty minutes to become aroused enough for good, orgasmic intercourse. If he wants to get on with the main event, but she's not ready, she can hold his penis still and stroke him everywhere else. This will desensitise him so he lasts longer. Delayed gratification means stronger orgasms.

Don't be afraid to be heavy-handed when handling a man: men have thicker skin than women. She can hold his balls in the palm of her hand and roll them around.

Instead of caressing her with his hands, he can use his breath. Less is more: his hot breath on her inner thighs, neck or stomach, clitoris and anus, is warm, intimate and arousing – and, unlike manual stimulation, he can never be too heavy-handed.

She knows you love playing with her breasts, but don't dive straight for them: women complain that men often spend the whole time jiggling the boobies and forgetting about the rest of the body. Instead, leave her sex organs for as long as she can bear it – if you feel like teasing her, maybe even a little bit longer. The anticipation means they'll be flushed, sensitive and far more responsive to touch.

He can use the tip of his penis to caress her and trace the outline of her vulva and clitoris. It's softer than his hands and leaves them free to touch her everywhere else.

SOLO WORKOUTS:
WHY MASTURBATION IS THE BEST MEDICINE

Think of **masturbation** – the act of stimulating yourself to orgasm – as the training in between matches. Research shows that people who masturbate regularly, whether they're single or in a relationship, are more aware of their body's sexual response systems and more able to communicate their needs to their partners. Plus, the more you masturbate, the more orgasms you have – and orgasms are shown to have very real health benefits for both men and women.

SOLO SEX FOR THE BOYS

We know that men don't need to be told how to masturbate, but did you know it's actually very good for you? Ejaculation flushes the toxins from your prostate gland, meaning you're less likely to get prostate cancer in the long-term.

As well as being a good way to pass the time while she's out shopping, masturbating can actually make you a better, longer-lasting lover. This will take a degree of re-training, because when you started to explore masturbation you were just trying to climax as quickly as possible: teenage boys tend to race towards the orgasm, partly because it feels nice and partly because they never know how long their privacy is

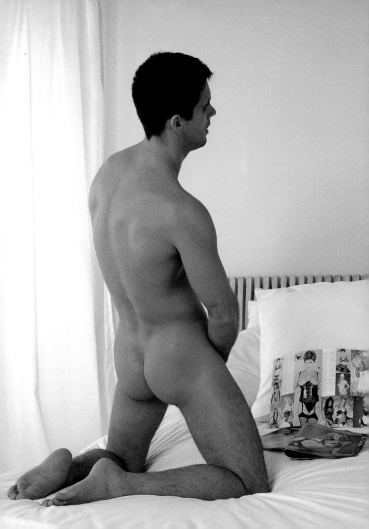

going to last! But changing the way you stimulate yourself means you can train yourself to last longer and delay your climax – thus increasing the time you can spend stimulating your lover, and upping her chances of having an orgasm.

Next time you masturbate, concentrate on the job (quite literally) in hand.

As you approach your climax, be aware of every change in your body. Learn to recognise the signs that mean you're about to reach your point of no return (that moment when you know you're going to come and there's nothing you can do about it). Just before you reach that point, stop touching yourself for a moment or two. The second you feel your erection begin to subside start stimulating yourself again, and stop just before you're about to cross the finishing line. This will take a while to perfect, but keep it up for as long as you can bear, and within a couple of months you should be able to last twice as long and stop three or four times during intercourse.

Transfer your skills by pulling out of her or lying still inside her vagina while you're having sex: use your 'downtime' to play with her breasts or clitoris. She'll be impressed at your new-found stamina and the extra attention you're able to pay her.

GIRLS ALONE

Let's get one thing straight: when it comes to masturbation, nice girls do. And smart girls do it quite a lot, actually. Women who are able to stimulate themselves to orgasm have a built-in stress-relief mechanism: regular orgasms, whether you get them solo or with a partner actually raise your immune system, so think of a little self-administered sex as a vitamin pill.

It used to be thought that it was possible to get addicted to masturbation, but the opposite is true: a woman who knows what turns her on is more likely to seek out good sex with a considerate partner. Once you can do it yourself, you can train him to give you a helping hand!

If you've never masturbated before, make sure you've got peace and quiet. Lie back in a bed or chair with your legs apart. Use a mirror to locate your clitoris if you're new to this – it's the little bud just above your urethra (where you pee). It should feel more sensitive to the touch than the rest of your vulva. Gently stroke it, experimenting with different techniques. Many women find that the clitoris is so sensitive it's uncomfortable to touch directly and prefer to use their fingers to make swirling, circling motions on the surrounding skin.

Read an erotic novel or fantasise about your favourite movie star or a friend you've always fancied. Let your thoughts and your hands run wild. Use some lubrication to ease your fingers over your clitoris but not so much that you can't feel the friction between your fingers and your genitals. Don't put any pressure on yourself: if the earth doesn't move tonight, try it again tomorrow, maybe this time kneeling or lying on your front.

Alternatively, use a warm jet of water in the shower to stimulate your clitoris: the consistent rhythm of the water is just the slow, steady stimulation women need to reach orgasm. However, it's not a good idea to direct the shower directly up your vagina as hot soapy water can upset the delicate balance of bacteria inside you.

When you've trained yourself to climax using your own hands, experiment with a vibrator, dildo or strap-on toy, but don't get too dependent on your battery-powered friend as some experts say that women who rely on vibrators become desensitised and unable to reach orgasm through manual stimulation. In the gym, you vary your workout to stop getting bored and keep you on your toes – the same principle must apply to masturbation!

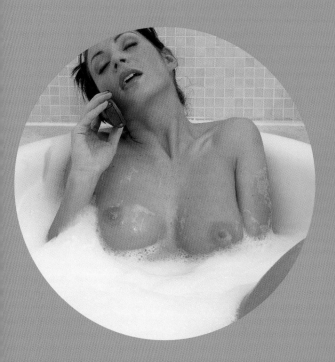

FOOD OF LOVE

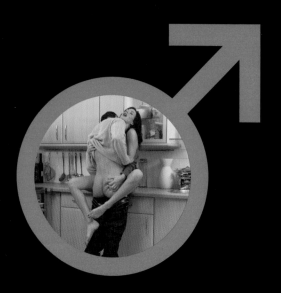

FOOD OF LOVE:
HOW TO EAT RIGHT FOR YOUR SEX LIFE

Food is big news right now. There are plenty of books to tell you how the right diet can improve your mood, body shape and energy levels, but did you know that the food you eat can also have a massive impact on your sex life? Athletes know that what they put in their body is just as important as the exercise they do. And the same is true when it comes to making love: eating the right stuff means you'll look better, your circulation will improve and your skin will respond better to touch, you'll smell and taste delicious and, if you're trying for a baby, you'll also be more fertile. Plus, avoiding the wrong stuff means you won't feel sluggish or bloated – qualities that aren't high on anyone's sex wish list.

It's not a coincidence that most foods that are reputed to have **aphrodisiac** properties – to excite sexual desire when eaten or drunk – are highly nutritious, too. They're also natural, simple and extremely tasty. Fresh fruit and vegetables balance hormones, flush out toxins and oxidise our blood so that energy levels are high and skin glows. They can also enrich your sex life when used creatively: hide a grape somewhere on your body and challenge your lover to find it using only his tongue.

Aim to eat at least five portions of fruit and veg a day. You should also fill up on foods containing essential fatty acids and B vitamins, which balance and regulate your hormones, such as oily fish, nuts and seaweeds. You need 45-plus nutrients daily to maintain good health (and therefore good orgasms), so if you can't eat well every day, it's also worth taking a multivitamin pill.

THE GOOD GUYS:
FOODS TO MAKE YOU GO MMMM ...

Bananas

No, not just because they're shaped like the male appendage (in fact, 'banana' is Spanish slang for penis). Bananas contain a substance called bufotenine that lifts the spirits and helps with self-confidence – always a good idea when you plan to get naked with someone. They're also rich in carbohydrate, so they boost your energy, which is good for **sexual stamina**. Munching on a banana prior to making love in a very energetic, demanding position is a good idea as they also contain potassium, which can help to ease muscle cramps.

Chocolate

Hurrah! Finally you've got an excuse for your hardcore Toblerone habit. Cocoa – the active ingredient in chocolate – increases mood-enhancing chemicals in your brain, especially phenylethylamine (PEA), dubbed the 'molecule of love' by sex researchers because it gives you a confidence buzz and makes you **ready for anything** in the bedroom. Chocolate also stimulates the production of endorphins, that fuzzy happy glow you get when you've just had an orgasm or when you're in love. Dark chocolate is better than milk as it contains more pure cocoa and less of the sugar and milk fats that can make you sluggish. Plus, anything that melts in the mouth is a sensual feast that just invites a lover's kiss ...

Fennel

Fennel contains estragole, the plant form of oestrogen, the female hormone. This means it's great for menopausal women

who want to boost their **libido** and women who want to
return to lovemaking after childbirth. It's also rumoured
to help strengthen male erections.

Olive oil

You might not be a virgin any more, but your olive oil should be!
Extra-virgin olive oil is rich in Vitamin E, often called the **sex
vitamin**, because it improves oxygen supply to the blood and
boosts testosterone production. It also plumps up skin, making
it softer and more sensitive. Although olive oil is high in calories,
it is a much healthier option than animal fats such as butter.

Nuts

Every vegetarian's favourite snack, nuts contain **selenium**, and
a deficiency of this mineral is linked with a low sex drive. Brazil
nuts are the richest in selenium. Nuts also contain nitric oxide
which promotes blood flow to the genitals (he gets a better
hard-on: she gets wetter).

Ginger

Fresh root ginger literally spices up your sex life as it's warming
and **stimulating**. It flushes out your digestive system so you're
wide awake, boosts your circulation and makes you more
sensitive to touch.

Oysters

Perhaps the most famous **aphrodisiac**, but no-one agrees
why. Some say it's because of their high zinc content, which
is important for male potency: he loses lots of zinc when
he ejaculates. Others insist it's because the salty taste and
marine smell are reminiscent of female genitalia. The fact

that they're an expensive delicacy and ideal for feeding
to each other makes them sensual and romantic.

Nutmeg
As well as counteracting a **low libido**, nutmeg can help with
nervous disorders and depression, so it's perfect for anyone
who finds their sex drive wanes when they've got the blues.
Grate fresh nutmeg onto your breakfast, but go easy – it can
be toxic in high quantities.

Honey
Honey contains bee pollen, which the ancient Greeks believed
gave them energy and increased their **sex drive**. Use it instead
of sugar to sweeten everyday foods. It's also an antiseptic and
great skin softener – oh, and it tastes delicious too.

Peaches
The ancient Chinese believed the peach to be an aphrodisiac
as its sensual shape, soft skin and abundant juices are evocative
of a young, **fertile** female body.

Champagne
Champagne goes hand-in-hand with oysters and is just as
luxurious. It has no real nutritional value, but a single glass
will lower your **sexual inhibitions** just enough to try out a
demanding new position. However, don't drain the bottle:
one glass is enough to raise testosterone levels (and therefore
sexual desire) but any more, and testosterone levels plummet
and you risk dehydration and a lack of sensation. Try kissing
with the bubbles in your mouth, or dribbling traces of the
sparkling wine over each other's chest and belly.

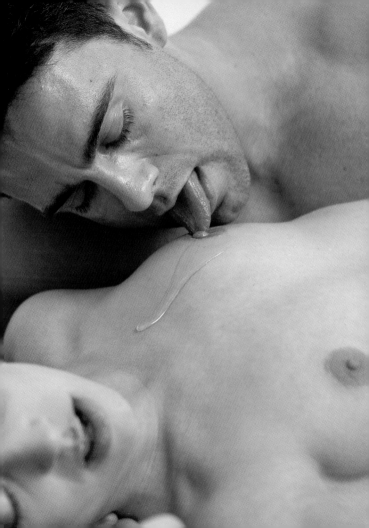

Vanilla

This creamy spice is a **strong aphrodisiac**, although some find the reason why rather unappetizing – apparently, it's the closest natural smell to our mother's breast milk, and takes us back to a vulnerable, affectionate stage in our lives.

THE BAD GUYS: FOODS TO AVOID

As well as those sexy foods that boost your love life, there are substances that can reduce libido and adversely affect your performance in bed. Avoiding the bad stuff is almost as important as stocking up on the good stuff: the following indulgences might seem like a good idea at the time, but consumed regularly they will depress your sex drive and inhibit your performance. Remember, a long-term slump in libido could affect your self-esteem and your relationship.

Alcohol

Booze stokes desire but it takes away the performance (see Champagne, page 46). After four units – that's two large glasses of wine, or two pints of beer – brewer's droop rears its ugly head, or rather, his penis doesn't, and the result is an erection that points downwards and is too floppy to penetrate properly. Some experts even claim alcohol decreases the size of the penis and testicles, although this is controversial. What is widely acknowledged is that excessive amounts can cause fertility problems and even impotence! Alcohol doesn't enhance lovemaking for her, either: she may become dehydrated and find it harder to lubricate, so sex might be painful and the risk of STIs increases as the tender skin around her vulva is more vulnerable. It also goes without saying that drunken lovers are much less likely to remember to use condoms.

Smoking

The post-coital cigarette is a movie cliché, but there's nothing sexy about smoking. Everyone knows that cigarettes cause fatal illnesses but in the short-term they can really stub out your sex life. Cigarettes depress the sex drive, lower a woman's oestrogen levels and can bring early menopause and infertility. Male smokers can suffer low sperm count and erectile dysfunction as the blood struggles to get around the body. And if you're both out of breath, you won't be able to attempt some of the more advanced positions in this book.

Sugar

Eating too many sweets, biscuits and processed foods (as opposed to the posh chocolate and organic honey mentioned above) can deplete levels of chromium and vitamin B. This drains your energy and makes your circulation sluggish.

Caffeine

Tea, cola drinks and coffee deplete zinc and magnesium when taken in excess, plus they strip the calcium from your bones. A single cup of coffee before sex has, however, been proven to make for an energetic bedroom experience – just don't forget the breath mints.

Drugs: what the doctor ordered

If your sex drive has dipped lately and you don't know why, think about any medication you're taking. Many prescription drugs, like the oral contraceptive pill, anti-depressants, hayfever remedies or painkillers can suppress your nervous system or alter your mood so you're not up for it. Talk to your doctor about any problems you're having.

Drugs: what the doctor didn't order

When you take drugs recreationally you don't know what you're getting into. Your nervous system will inevitably be affected, slowing down your body's natural sexual responses. Marijuana slows the body's reflexes and dulls sensation (your mind may be racing, but your body's a blob). Many people take ecstasy as it heightens sensations and intimacy, but as no long-term research has been done experts are concerned that in the long term your body might lose the ability to naturally produce feel-good hormones such as serotonin. Likewise, cocaine might feel good in the very short term but it is addictive and in the long term can stop your body's ability to produce dopamine, leading to depression and impotence.

ON THE MENU

Obviously, a dedicated sexerciser eats well all the time, but why not experiment by eating **smart foods** – meals created with specific sexual needs in mind? Big, rich meals eaten just before sex can make you feel lethargic and less likely to experiment, but food with specially selected aphrodisiac ingredients will leave you satisfied but light, energetic and oh-so-horny.

The ritual of sharing food with a lover is as important as the food itself: there's a reason why dinner *à deux* is the most popular first date. As well as preparing these meals, decorate the table or have an indoor picnic by spreading the tablecloth over the floor and decorating with rose petals. Use colour, aroma and soft music to add to your gastronomic experience. *Bon appetit*!

Before quickie sex . . .

A hot drink of lemon, ginger and honey gives you a tingly circulation boost to intensify your lover's kisses and caresses. You can buy ready-made infusions, but for maximum benefit grate some fresh root ginger, squeeze a slice of lemon and dribble some organic honey into a glass of boiling water. Kissing with the warm liquid in your mouth will make foreplay even more delicious than usual.

Before tantric sex . . .

If you plan on a long, drawn-out sex session, you need to eat slow-release carbohydrates that will keep hunger pangs at bay (nothing interrupts the flow of deep spiritual bonding like having to get up for a bagel halfway through). A bowl of porridge with blueberries is a clean, healthy start to the day that will give you the energy you need to go on, and on, and on. Also great before lazy Sunday-morning sex.

Before oral sex . . .

You are what you eat is never truer than during oral sex: your sex juices (semen if you're a man; vaginal lubrication if you're a woman) literally take on the flavour of the foods you've consumed over the last day or so. If you're going to attempt the simultaneous oral sex positions on pages 70–72, it pays to lay off the rich, spicy foods for a couple of days and treat yourselves to fruit salads made with chopped mangoes, melon, strawberries, apples and pears. This mixture will also have a detoxing effect, so your body will be zinging with energy as well as lust.

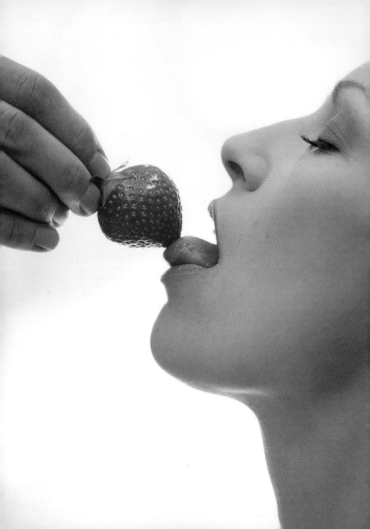

Before afternoon sex . . .

There's nothing more luxurious than sex in the afternoon when everyone (including you) should really be at work. Set yourselves up for great sex with a tricolor salad of sliced avocado, tomato and mozzarella. Avocado was thought to represent a man's testicles in ancient Greece, and it is rich in essential fatty acids. Add beef tomatoes, which contain lypocene, which protects against prostate cancer, and low-fat mozzarella for a sensual oral treat. Scatter with torn fresh basil, which is said to promote wellbeing and sexual energy, and season with balsamic vinegar and a dash of pepper to bring out the fiery, passionate Mediterranean in you!

Before snuggled-up-by-the-fire sex . . .

Spaghetti with caviar is a warming treat perfect for sharing on a winter's evening: every main ingredient is an aphrodisiac, and spaghetti is the perfect sensual treat to accompany this rich, sexy sauce. While the pasta's boiling, heat butter, cream, chopped cooked asparagus and smoked salmon in a saucepan. Stir the cooked pasta in, top with just a dash of caviar and serve at once. Tip: spaghetti is notorious for staining clothes. So you'd better turn up the heat and eat it in your underwear!

Before special-occasion sex . . .

Chocolate-dipped strawberries are the ultimate in luxury aphrodisiacs and are surprisingly easy to make. You can buy chocolate fondue sets in department stores, but melting a bar of high-cocoa chocolate in a heatproof bowl placed over a saucepan of hot water will do. Using skewers, dip the strawberries into the melted chocolate and feed them to each other. Or, if you're feeling creative, use the strawberries to write rude suggestions on your lover's flesh: if he doesn't carry out your dare, he doesn't get any more strawberries!

During sex!
Baked figs were a Roman aphrodisiac: for a modern twist, drizzle them with melted butter and bake them for 30 minutes at 200°C/400°F/gas mark 6. Serve with vanilla ice cream, lashings of honey and the syrupy juices from the bottom of the jar. Feed it to each other from a bowl or serve it from your bodies: your flesh will love the hot-and-cold sensation of this dish and it will really wake up your nerve endings, making every touch more intense.

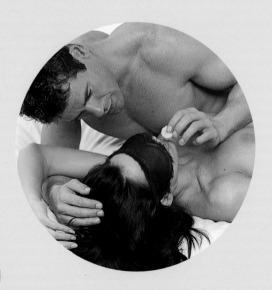

POSITIONS

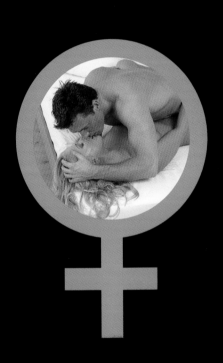

ALL THE RIGHT MOVES: POSITIONS THAT GET RESULTS IN MORE WAYS THAN ONE

These hot sex positions tone specific body parts AND produce fabulous orgasms. They can be done as part of foreplay before assuming your favourite position, or as the main event. Try them with your clothes on for a fun workout. We've rated each one for difficulty and required fitness levels – common sense will tell you which to avoid if you or your partner are too heavy, as they might exacerbate any injuries you already have. If you're pregnant, don't attempt any but the easiest positions.

Vary your sexperiences: try these positions immediately after exercise to make the most of your increased circulation, energy levels and those delicious pheromones. Once you've mastered your favourite, why not incorporate one of our deliciously kinky, exercise-themed twists?

THE FLING

How to do it: From a kneeling position, she lies on her back with her legs folded under her thighs so her pelvis is elevated. She flings her arms above her head while he lies on top of her and enters her. She can hang her head back over the edge of the bed while he uses his upper arms to bear his body weight and moves his whole body, grinding his pelvis into her clitoris, which works his buttocks too.

What's in it for him? This enables really deep thrusting, plus his hands are free to explore erogenous zones that aren't always accessible during intercourse, such as her underarms

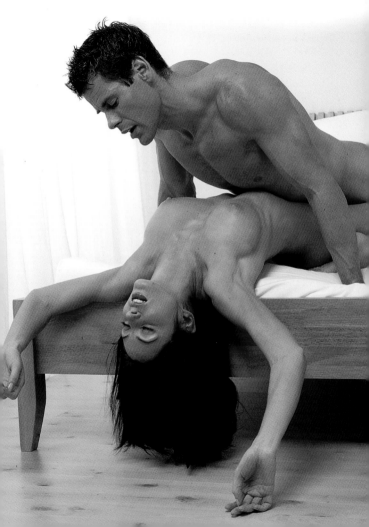

and sides. Her intense vulnerability – she can't go anywhere, trapped by his bodyweight – can be a massive turn-on, too.
Stamina: 3   Strength: 3   Flexibility: 3   Orgasmability: 4

What's in it for her? Her clitoris is clamped between his penis and the hard surface of her flexed ab muscles, meaning it's stimulated from all angles. This is a great stretch for her legs, and she's free to lean back as little or as much as she wants to maximise the stretch in her legs and control the depth of penetration. If she's very fit (or wildly ambitious) she can work a stomach crunch into this move, raising her upper body towards his for a stolen kiss.
Stamina: 4   Strength: 4   Flexibility: 4   Orgasmability: 4

Sexercise twist: Try some role-play games while making love in this position to experiment with notions of power and obedience (after all, the mind is a very powerful erogenous zone). Perhaps he's a demanding personal trainer, and she's the bored, rich housewife who longs to be dominated and ordered around. He can dress up in sports gear while she remains naked but for her jewellery, to help the fantasy come alive.

THIGH MISTRESS

How to do it: He lies on his back, but she's doing all the work, so he's free to sink back into the pillows and enjoy watching her work out! She straddles him and gently slides down onto his erection, with her feet flat on the bed at either side of his body. She then uses her thighs to move up and down his erection, pulling out as far as she can comfortably go.

This is all about control – she can vary the pace according to the effects her stimulation is having on him. Using her PC muscles, she can draw his penis as far out of the body as it can go before it pops out. This stimulates the tip of his penis and the sensitive opening of her vagina. For maximum effect, she should do nine shallow thrusts and bear right down on him at the tenth, plunging as deep onto his penis as she can.

What's in it for him? This is a real treat for the guy, not just visually, but because he expends very little energy. Sexual etiquette demands that he stimulates her clitoris if that's what she needs to tip her over the edge into orgasm – after all, she's working really hard up there!
Stamina: 1   Strength: 1   Flexibility: 1   Orgasmability: 4

What's in it for her? This is great for women with an exhibitionist, dominating streak. She controls everything, from the depth of the penetration to the pace of the thrusting. Plus, he's helpless and vulnerable beneath her, which can be a real turn-on. This is a great workout for her butt, thighs and PC muscles but can be too demanding to sustain for longer than a few minutes. If she's getting tired, she can rest on him for a while, using her PC muscles to keep stimulating his penis, while both lovers pay attention to her breasts and clitoris.
Stamina: 4   Strength: 4   Flexibility: 2   Orgasmability: 4

Sexercise twist: To increase her feeling of empowerment and strength (and to build up her upper body), she can try this position while clutching a pair of dumbbells. She can't touch him, which makes him crave her hands on his skin even more. Trust is everything in this game, and she can toy with his feelings of vulnerability. She wouldn't drop the weights on him, would she? It can be incredibly liberating for men – who often feel they have to be the dominant, 'active' partner during sex – to surrender like this.

CARRY ON COMING

How to do it: She stands facing away from him and he enters her from behind. Once penetration is established, he circles one arm around her stomach and grabs hold of her leg with the other. She then carefully lifts her legs behind her so he's supporting her and gently rocks her way to orgasm. Balancing is hard and you'll both tire easily. Get around this by indulging in lots of foreplay first so you're both on the brink of orgasm before you assume the position.

What's in it for him? This is the most physically demanding position in the book for men: he needs to be strong enough to bear her entire weight (which means she needs to be reasonably light).
Stamina: 5   Strength: 5   Flexibility: 3   Orgasmability: 3

What's in it for her? This is also one of the hardest positions for her to assume, but worth it if her idea of heaven is to be supported by a strong, sexy lover. If fatigue takes over before you're ready, she can lean over and place her hands on the floor – this takes stress away from her core muscles and legs, and instead gives her an upper body workout, while it relieves the pressure on him.
Stamina: 5   Strength: 4   Flexibility: 5   Orgasmability: 3

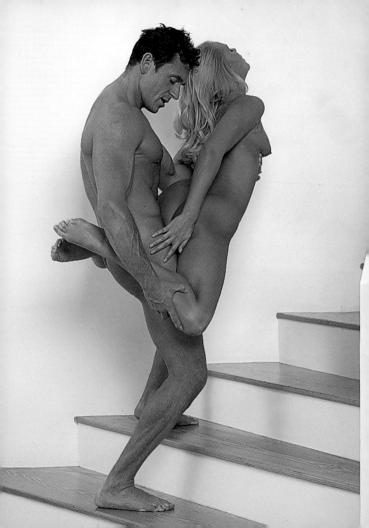

Sexercise twist: Most gyms have a mirrored wall in which muscle men can admire themselves. This exhibitionist position demands an audience, even if it's just the two of you, so face a full-length mirror and watch yourselves enjoying the contortions. Some people find that rear-entry sex is impersonal as you can't see each other's faces, but this solves that problem as you can lock eyes with your partner's mirror image as you bounce to a climax.

STANDING DOGGY

How to do it: He needs a full erection. She stands facing away from him leaning against a wall or holding onto something like a window sill or bed-end for support. He gets behind her and bends his legs until he's low enough to penetrate her from the rear. Both bend your legs until you've found a position you're comfortable with, and gently bounce your way to a climax. This one takes some getting used to, so if she finds it hard to balance, she can bend over until she feels confident enough to stand up. If there's a discrepancy in height, she could stand on a step or the edge of a bed.

What's in it for him? Her closed legs act as an extension of the vagina, making for tighter penetration for him and stimulating the nerve endings on her labia and inner thighs. He uses the muscle groups in his legs, which burn lots of calories, and he'll need upper body strength to help her balance.

Stamina: 4   Strength: 4   Flexibility: 3   Orgasmability: 4

What's in it for her? The gentle, bouncing motion uses tiny movements to tone her legs and butt: this is very effective, but she must stretch beforehand or she risks cramp. This is the perfect position if she's got very long, lean legs or is the taller partner.

Stamina: 4   Strength: 4   Flexibility: 4   Orgasmability: 3

Sexercise twist: Slipping into a pair of salsa-dancing stilettos will make a difference to both partners. It lengthens her legs, making them appear even more toned and sexy, and tips the angle of her hips slightly forward so that penetration is tighter for both of you. Plus, because her heels are raised, she's toning a completely different set of leg muscles.

LIFT OFF!

How to do it: He begins kneeling and asks her to lower herself onto his erection, facing him. As she does, she wraps her legs around his waist and puts her arms up around his neck. Then he slowly stands up, so that he's holding her in his arms, and slowly rocks and bounces her to a climax that will have her seeing stars.

What's in it for him? His arms in particular receive a vigorous workout. It takes all his reserves of strength to bear her weight for the time it takes to climax. This can mean he doesn't have the energy to reach orgasm himself: which can be useful if he suffers from premature ejaculation, but frustrating if his arms give up before his penis gives out!

Stamina: 5   Strength: 5   Flexibility: 3   Orgasmability: 3

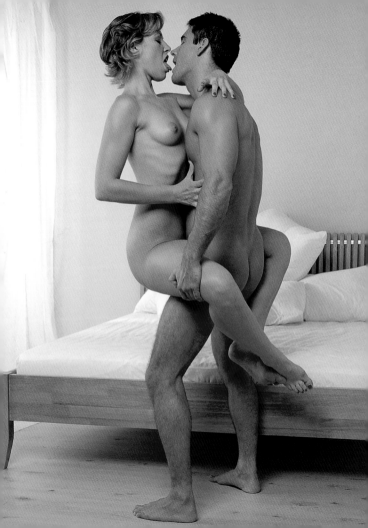

What's in it for her? Every woman likes her man to pick her up and carry her: even though he's bearing her weight, her limbs, which are wrapped around her lover, will be toned as she uses them to keep her balance. Although neither of them have their hands free to stimulate her clitoris, the full-body friction of her breasts rubbing against his chest and her clitoris grinding against his pubic bone should get her off.

Stamina: 5   Strength: 4   Flexibility: 4   Orgasmability: 4

Sexercise twist: Get aquabatic: doing this position in a swimming pool means your muscles will be supported by the water: you can concentrate on the sensations you're feeling rather than using your strength to support each other. Plus, the slippery wet sensations of the water and the gentle splashing motions will caress your skin like hundreds of tiny hands. Just make sure the lifeguard's back is turned!

THE KICK INSIDE

How to do it: Begin as with missionary sex: she lies back on the bed while he climbs on top of her. She opens and closes her legs during sex, so that viewed from above, she looks like a pair of scissors opening and closing. She can spread her legs as wide as they'll go, giving her legs a good workout and creating an interesting range of sensations for both partners. Closing the legs makes it easier to clench thigh muscles, and this stimulates the inner clitoris, the nerve endings of which actually reach all the way down to the thighs and up to the stomach. Although she's doing a lot of small movements, this is a comparatively low-effort position with powerful results.

What's in it for him? Although he's on top, he doesn't have to put much effort in besides using his elbows to prop himself up and making sure he doesn't squash her. As with all man-on-top positions, the clenching of his butt when he climaxes will help tone and define his rear end.

Stamina: 3   Strength: 3   Flexibility: 3   Orgasmability: 5

What's in it for her? As well as stimulating the inner clitoris, this position creates delicious sensations on her outer genitals. Opening and closing creates friction on the outer, visible part of the clitoris, and the inner folds of the vulva, which are rich in nerve bundles. She can control the speed and strength of her leg movements, which in turn provide a great inner thigh workout – a problem area for most women.

Stamina: 3   Strength: 3   Flexibility: 3   Orgasmability: 5

Sexercise twist: Get creative with dynabands, the rubber ribbons that you use to help you stretch in the gym. If she ties her feet together with a band, she has much more resistance and her legs will receive a far better workout. This is great for those who haven't tried bondage but are curious to experiment, as the soft rubber won't hurt the skin, and there's plenty of room for movement. Tying her hands to the bedpost so she's utterly at his mercy will take this power-and-surrender game to another, wonderful level . . .

WHEELBARROW

How to do it: She begins on all fours either on the floor or a bed. He carefully takes hold of her ankles and raises them until they are level with his hips, so her hands are the only part of her body on the floor and her pelvis is in mid-air. The man lifts her legs up and holds them spread apart as he penetrates her from behind. The woman can also wrap her legs around the man's waist (crossing her ankles behind her back) for extra support. This position requires upper body strength from both of you. If it's too wobbly, try leaning your upper body on a bed or chair rather than trying to support your whole body with your arms. Just make sure she has a pillow placed under her breasts to absorb some of the shock of the vigorous thrusting.

What's in it for him? It gives the man a nice view of his partner's backside and works most of the major muscle groups, particularly his back, arms, thighs and glutes. Although it looks as if he's doing a lot of work, once penetration is achieved, it's relatively easy to thrust his way to orgasm so long as she can keep her balance.
Stamina: 3   Strength: 4   Flexibility: 3   Orgasmability: 4

What's in it for her? Like all rear-entry positions, the Wheelbarrow stimulates her G-spot. Her breasts will jiggle about a lot, and even if he can't see it happening, it means that the blood flows to them so that her nipples will be ultra-sensitive to the touch if you then decide to swap to a face-to-face position. If she has any issues about her body, particularly her ass, she might feel a bit vulnerable and exposed. She has

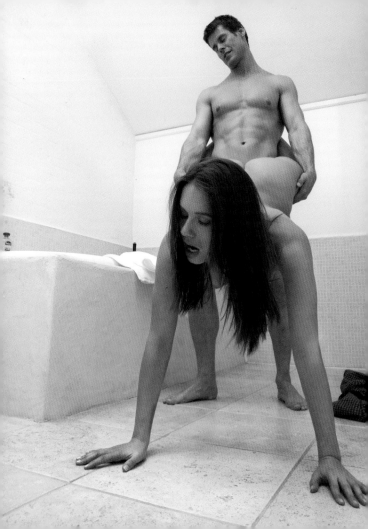

to trust him not to drop her as well – if she's worrying about him bearing her weight, she won't climax.

Stamina: 4   Strength: 4   Flexibility: 4   Orgasmability: 4

Sexercise twist: He can increase the intensity of his experience (and his workout) by attaching weights to his ankles and wrists. As he works harder, his body temperature rises, causing his testosterone levels to rise too – meaning he can carry on in this position for longer.

LAPDANCE

How to do it: He sits in an armchair while she straddles him, with her legs hanging over either side of his lap. She can relax while he uses his thigh and PC muscles to push his penis deep inside her. If she starts to squash him, she can place her toes on the floor and gently bounce up and down in time to his thrusting movements. If she's much smaller than him, or her legs don't reach the floor, she can place her feet on the side of the chair instead.

What's in it for him? Although he's expending lots of energy by controlling the penetration and bearing her weight, he's sitting down so shouldn't tire easily. He might find it takes longer than usual for him to climax as the blood will be pumping to the muscles around his penis, which means there's less blood in his penis to tip him over the edge into orgasm. This is good news for her as it gives him more time to stimulate her clitoris, and her breasts are at the perfect level for him to kiss and caress.

Stamina: 3   Strength: 4   Flexibility: 2   Orgasmability: 3

What's in it for her? The face-to-face intimacy and full-body friction will drive her wild. He can put his hands on her waist, a nice touch which makes her feel vulnerable in what can seem like an aggressive position.

Stamina: 3   Strength: 3   Flexibility: 3   Orgasmability: 3

Sexercise twist: Instead of sitting on an armchair, try this position balanced on a Swiss exercise ball. You use your legs, abs and back to balance so you'll both get a full-body workout. Many people find the sweaty, slippery feeling of bare skin on the rubber of the ball a sensual turn-on. You'll probably fall off the first couple of times you try, so this one's for lovers with a sense of humour as well as balance!

69, MAN ON TOP

How to do it: Giving and receiving oral sex at the same time is a fantasy many of us never realise as the logistics are quite complicated – it can feel more like a game of Twister than a loving exchange – but this position is the easiest way to achieve mutual bliss with the guy taking control. She lies back on the bed, legs slightly parted, arms by her side. He crouches over her on all fours and is in an excellent position to play with her breasts. This is a comfortable position for him because his neck won't start to ache. He can also use her inner thighs as a pillow.

What's in it for him? It's not easy for the woman to take him fully into her mouth from this angle, but he can thrust against her neck, cheeks and breasts and she's free to use her tongue

on his anus, balls and perineum (the super-sensitive piece
of skin between his balls and anus).
Stamina: 4   Strength: 4   Flexibility: 5   Orgasmability: 4

What's in it for her? If she spreads her legs as wide as
she can, the skin surrounding the clitoris and vagina will
be stretched tight, leaving it more exposed and sensitive,
and giving him a unique close-up look at her genitals. He
can also pay attention to the inner thighs, an often-neglected
erogenous zone. He can see exactly what he's doing so
there's no excuse for him not finding her clitoris and paying
it lots of attention with his tongue!
Stamina: 3   Strength: 3   Flexibility: 5   Orgasmability: 4

Sexercise twist: Take this session into the bathroom. Turn
up the heat, run the hot tap and make love in the steam on
the bathroom floor (if she lies on a fluffy towel she will be
much more comfortable). Pretend that you're two strangers
who have been looking at each other across a crowded gym
and who just happened to follow each other to the sauna . . .
the steam in the room will bring everything into soft-focus,
meaning it's easy to assume other identities.

69, WOMAN ON TOP

How to do it: This is the most common 69 position for the
simple reason that women tend to be lighter than men. He
lies flat on his back with his arms by his sides or around her
buttocks. She's on all fours with her bottom in the air, hovering
over his face. She rests on her forearms, her mouth poised

over his penis. It's hard to concentrate on giving head and getting it at the same time so take it in turns. Spend alternate minutes stimulating one another's genitals – this should build up to a tremendous orgasm for both of you. Or use it as foreplay and savour what you've just done while you're making love in a more conventional position.

What's in it for him? There's less work for his pleasure! His arms are free to caress her or to stimulate himself if she gets tired.
Stamina: 2   Strength: 2   Flexibility: 3   Orgasmability: 4

What's in it for her? She can control the rhythm of the cunnilingus she's receiving by rocking her hips in time and she's perfectly positioned to pay attention to every inch of his penis. Her breasts will brush against his belly and thighs, which will turn him on and the friction on her nipples will stimulate her, too. The twists and turns she makes during this position will stretch, loosen and lengthen her spine and limbs.
Stamina: 4   Strength: 4   Flexibility: 4   Orgasmability: 4

Sexercise twist: Why not listen to your favourite 'workout' CD? It can be hard to manage a steady rhythm when you're both giving and receiving at the same time. Loud, fast, pumping music means you can stimulate each other at a steady pace in time to the beat. The results of this position are so orgasmic that music has the added benefit of drowning out your moans of pleasure.

THE MEXICAN WAVE

How to do it: She lies on her back with her legs up in the air, open and wide apart. He lowers himself face down, facing away from her. His head is by her feet, and his legs are over her hips so his feet are on either side of her shoulders. She can rest her legs on his back or, for a super Sexercise twist, she can use her stomach muscles to keep them suspended in mid-air. She can play with his balls as he thrusts in and out of her. She can also hold onto his hips and pull herself up and towards him for an extra deep thrust that gives his penis and her vagina a delicious massage. Because you're only touching at the genital area, and your heads are as far away from each other as it's possible to be during intercourse, the sensations in your genitals are further intensified.

What's in it for him? This position works out his stomach, arms and thighs. He'll need a strong back as her feet, resting on his back, will put pressure on this part of his body. If he likes to have his ass played with, this is a prime position – although it will take an incredibly flexible partner to reach his anus with her mouth!
Stamina: 4   Strength: 4   Flexibility: 3   Orgasmability: 3

What's in it for her? When she extends her legs, the muscles in her lower abdomen and her PC muscles also contract. As well as having a fabulous toning effect, this also stimulates her inner clitoris, doubling her chances of orgasm.
Stamina: 3   Strength: 3   Flexibility: 3   Orgasmability: 3

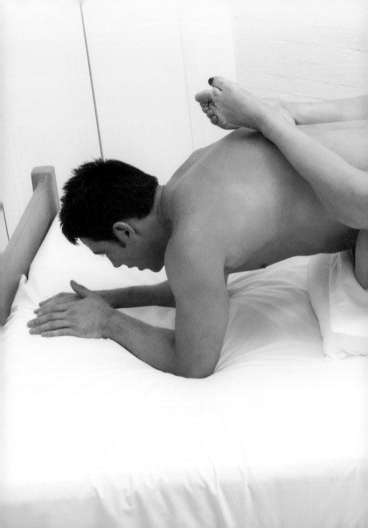

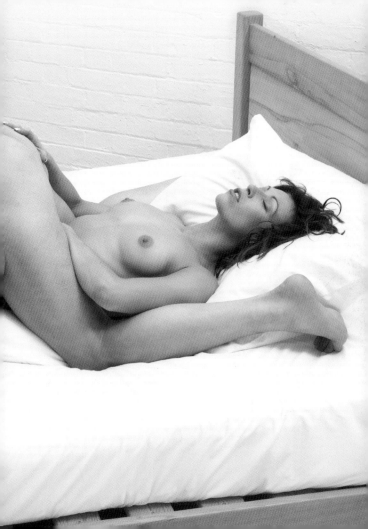

Sexercise twist: Blindfold each other using dynabands. You can't see each other anyway, but removing all vision means that your other senses – sight, sound, taste and smell – take over, and sex becomes a completely new experience. This position is one in which the sensations are already concentrated in the genitals. Blindfolding ups the intensity even further, making it a sexual experience you'll never forget.

THE CRUNCH

How to do it: He lies on his back. She straddles him and gently lowers herself onto his erection, with her legs tucked underneath her bottom. Instead of her controlling the movement with her thighs, he does sit-up-style moves that bring his upper body towards hers: he can punctuate each 'sit-up' with a bite of the nipples or a kiss on the lips. Each time he sits up, he slightly alters the angle of his erection inside her and the movement of his pelvic bone alters the friction on her clitoris. He can grab her waist or buttocks to help him balance. Start with one or two crunches and work up to ten or fifteen.

What's in it for him? This is a great opportunity for a man with strong, ripped abs to show off his body. The change in the angle of her vagina as he raises his body up means that his penis is constantly receiving different stimulation, so even though he can't thrust very much, he may climax sooner than usual.

Stamina: 5   Strength: 5   Flexibility: 5   Orgasmability: 5

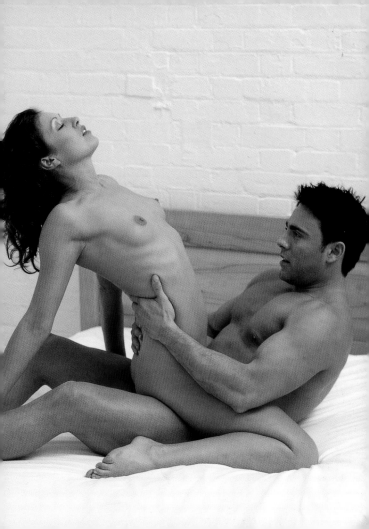

What's in it for her? She doesn't have to do much apart from bump and grind on his penis, and admire him as he sits up to meet her. It's important that she provides enough weight to stabilise his body. His eyes and mouth will be level with her breasts with every crunch he does – so she can enjoy short, sharp, intense kisses and nibbles on her nipples. Her hands are also free to stimulate her clitoris.

Stamina: 3   Strength: 3   Flexibility: 3   Orgasmability: 4

Sexercise twist: Do this one on a yoga or stretching mat: not only will it protect his spine against bruises, the smell and texture of the mat will make him feel he's really working out in the gym, and you're both free to fantasise that you're not really at home, but in a high-class spa with beautiful people watching you, fascinated by the way your bodies look together.

MIND,
BODY,
SPIRIT

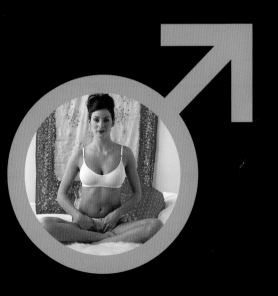

HOLISTIC SEX: MIND, BODY AND SPIRIT MOVES

The last ten years have seen a record number of health-conscious people realising that there's more to fitness than pumping iron and pounding the treadmill. The boom in disciplines like yoga, Pilates and T'ai Chi, which focus on holding poses and controlled breathing patterns, is proof that we want exercise that nourishes our spirit and soothes our minds as well as burning fat and toning the body.

The following positions are inspired by the *Kama Sutra*, the oldest and most famous sex manual in the world. It was written in the 4th Century BC by Prince Vatsyayana, who subscribed to the ancient Indian belief that sex was a way of attaining spiritual awareness, worshipping the gods and cleansing the soul. Using many of the same principles as yoga, these positions are just as sexually charged but the emphasis is on breathing in time with your partner and making a spiritual connection, rather than the fast, furious thrusting of more conventional Western sex. They are designed to delay the man's orgasm (and so conserve the sexual energy ancient Indians valued so highly) and intensify the female orgasm.

These mind, body and spirit moves require patience and flexibility rather than big muscles and raw lust – but bring physical and emotional rewards you never imagined possible. They don't burn as many calories as Western lovemaking, but are equally effective when it comes to toning specific body parts.

The *Kama Sutra* teaches that the mind and spirit are the most powerful tools in your sexual repertoire, so before attempting these positions, lie side by side and synchronise your breathing until you're breathing in time with each other. Try to empty your minds of all thoughts but those of your lover:

focus on a favourite body part, on your lover's face at the moment of climax, or a romantic experience you've shared. This helps you tune into each other's bodies and minds on a subtle but profound level. Instead of conventional foreplay, why not try the stretches-for-two on pages 23–26?

THE WIDELY OPENED POSITION

How to do it: Begin as though you were making love in the missionary position: he's on top, resting on his elbows, she's lying on her back. Once he's snugly inside her, she wraps her legs around his back, raising her pelvis as she does so, ensuring that her clitoris remains in contact with his pubic bone. He then rises up on all fours, so that he is bearing her whole bodyweight with his back and shoulders. He stays absolutely stationary while she rubs her clitoris against his pubic bone, making sure she gets the stimulation she needs to orgasm. This gives him just enough friction to maintain his erection, but not quite enough to cause him to climax. As she approaches orgasm, she can afford to arouse him a little more. If she pulls herself only halfway onto his penis, she focuses on the nerve endings in the super-sensitive tip of his penis. The widely opened position obviously depends on a reasonably light woman and a reasonably strong man who doesn't have any back problems.

What's in it for him? This is the equivalent of doing press-ups with weights strapped to the upper body: it requires strong arms, legs, back and shoulders but is excellent for building muscle. It's good for guys who suffer from premature ejaculation: the effort it takes him to carry her bodyweight

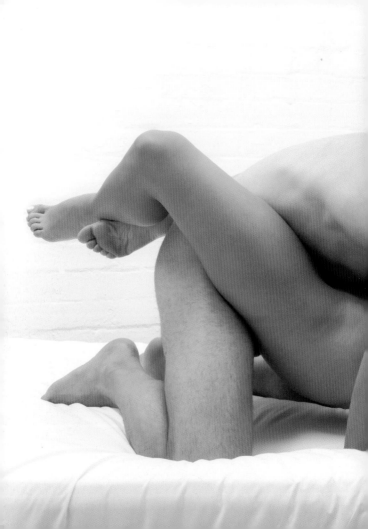

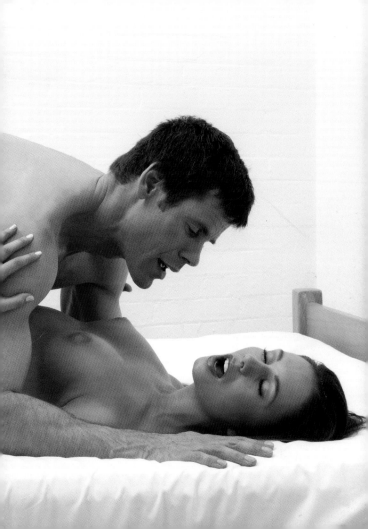

can buy precious extra minutes of intercourse as blood rushes away from his erection to his upper body muscles. However, he may miss the feeling of tight containment he gets when she closes her legs against his penis.

Stamina: 5   Strength: 5   Flexibility: 3   Orgasmability: 3

What's in it for her? Her legs need to be strong enough to stay wrapped around his waist for the duration of intercourse. Although he'll carry her bodyweight, she'll also need strong triceps, as her arms will inevitably bear much of her upper body. But after making love in this position she should notice an improvement in the muscle tone in her limbs. Orgasm-wise, this position gives her clitoris full exposure to the friction of intercourse and she controls that friction, meaning she can rub at a pace and intensity which suits her perfectly.

Stamina: 4   Strength: 4   Flexibility: 4   Orgasmability: 5

THE YAB-YUM

How to do it: He sits on the bed with his legs bent: she lowers herself onto his erection, wraps her arms and legs around him and slowly raises her legs over his shoulders. Instead of thrusting up and down, the woman clenches and unclenches her vaginal muscles, keeping up just enough pelvic movement to keep his penis erect inside her, but not so much that he feels he's approaching climax. When you've both reached orgasm, don't pull apart: satisfied, remain in the yab-yum position, breathing harmoniously until his penis is totally limp. We rarely allow this to happen, but it's a very gentle, intimate end to a lovemaking session.

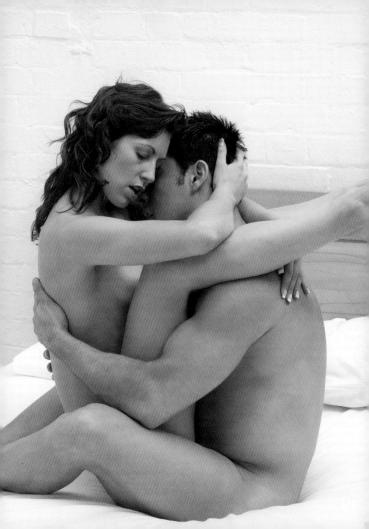

What's in it for him? A fantastic upper body workout: it takes all his reserves of strength to keep her upright while her legs are over his shoulders. Plus, Tantric practitioners believe that if a man's spine is erect during intercourse, he's able to moderate his passion and delay his ejaculation for up to six hours. That might be a little ambitious for those of us not schooled in the discipline, but he's not likely to suffer from premature ejaculation, and this is a fabulous position for letting him focus not on his own pleasure but on that of his partner.

Stamina: 4   Strength: 4   Flexibility: 3   Orgasmability: 3

What's in it for her? This offers her the deeper penetration she needs, while the top of her vagina is stretched and lengthened by this position, denying him the stimulation at the tip of the penis that might trip him over into premature climax. Her raised legs are also being stretched, making them appear longer and leaner. His upper body provides the perfect resistance for her to stretch against. And the vaginal squeezes are an excellent workout for her PC muscles.

Stamina: 3   Strength: 3   Flexibility: 4   Orgasmability: 4

THE ELEPHANT POSTURE

How to do it: This was inspired by the mating patterns of the elephants that roamed wild around India, which isn't the most obvious erotic image for modern lovers – however, the thrill of this position is timeless. She lies face-down with breasts stomach, thighs and feet all touching the bed. He lies over her with the small of his back arched inward. She raises her

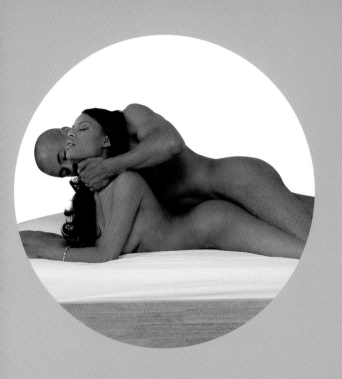

buttocks so that he can penetrate her – she might find
it easier to slip a pillow under her hips so that her bottom is
pointing upwards and he has a good view of her vagina when
she spreads her legs. Once he is inside her, the woman can
intensify the sensations for both partners by pressing her
thighs closely together.

What's in it for him? This is great for the man who likes to be in control. Penetration is snug and stimulates her G-spot. He supports himself using his arms, which works his upper body. His thighs and butt will contract as he pumps in and out of her. To give his hamstrings and calves an extra workout, he can bear his entire bodyweight on his toes.

Stamina: 4   Strength: 3   Flexibility: 2   Orgasmability: 5

What's in it for her? She doesn't get much of a workout during this position. In fact, she can barely move because of the depth of penetration and the weight of her lover bearing down on her. Many women find this total lack of control incredibly arousing, but it shouldn't be attempted if she suffers from claustrophobia.

Stamina: 4   Strength: 3   Flexibility: 2   Orgasmability: 4

KAMA'S WHEEL

How to do it: He sits with his legs outstretched and parted. She faces him and lowers herself onto his penis, extending her legs over his so that they point out past his back. His arms encircle her, supporting her upper back and her hands grasp the outside of his upper arms. Both partners lean back, creating the circular shape that gives this position its name. This position was originally about meditation rather than orgasm and isn't always erotically satisfying, but is worth trying as a warm-up. It can promote enormous feelings of intimacy and trust as you're both relying on each other to support your bodyweight.

What's in it for him? This position works most major muscle groups. His back and shoulders are working hard to support her weight as she leans back in his arms; as he leans back, his thighs will need to be strong to support his upper body. In terms of his sexual satisfaction, thrusting is almost impossible in this position: in fact, it's more of a meditation than a race towards a climax. It can be very liberating for a man to focus on intercourse when orgasm isn't the sole aim.

Stamina: 4   Strength: 5   Flexibility: 4   Orgasmability: 2

What's in it for her? Many women love the sense of surrender and vulnerability this position promotes: with her head flung back to expose her breasts and upper body, and her legs parted to reveal her clitoris and vulva, she can revel in the attention as her lover enjoys the view. She can use her stomach and back muscles to maintain her balance, and the stretch runs from the top of her head to the tips of her outstretched toes. Clitoral stimulation (and thefore orgasm) is unfortunately almost impossible without the aid of external stimulation like a strap-on vibrator.

Stamina: 4   Strength: 4   Flexibility: 2   Orgasmability: 1

COOLING DOWN

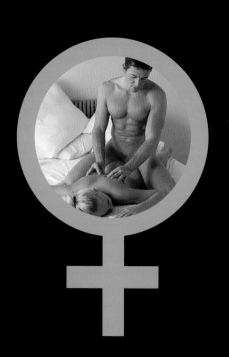

THE COOL-DOWN: POST-SEX RITUALS

After a big game, athletes have a hot bath and a massage
to ease them and their bodies back into real life. Why not
prolong your sexual experience with some of these **cooling-
down** techniques?

The right attitude to *après-sex* can make the difference
between good sex and great lovemaking. Afterplay is especially
important after quickie sex where you've been too charged to
linger over foreplay. Pillow talk and stroking as you come down
from the high of your orgasm can bring an emotional intimacy
to what was a highly physical event.

A PAMPERING SPA

Anyone who's ever slipped into a hot bath to relax aching
muscles after a big workout or sporting event will tell you that
nothing beats hot water when it comes to pampering and
relaxing . . . so why not turn your bathroom into a spa and get
hot and steamy together? Pay attention to your surroundings.
Keep the health-and-fitness theme going through your afterplay.
Even if your bathroom isn't up to professional spa standards,
some fresh, white fluffy towels will introduce an air of
cleanliness, health and efficiency to rival any designer wetroom.

Run the shower as hot as possible, steaming up the
bathroom. The steam will cleanse your pores and get rid of
impurities as well as enhancing your flushed, sultry, post-sex
glow. Write erotic messages for each other on the steamed-up
bathroom mirror. Get into the shower and wash each other all
over with an unscented soap so that your genitals, still sensitive,
aren't irritated. If you have a power shower, hold the jet of water
against each other's shoulders and buttocks, and any other
parts of the body that have taken the strain during your

energetic lovemaking session! Finally, take a tip from the Swiss, who roll in the snow after a hot sauna – finish off with a blast of icy cold water to close your pores, tone up your muscles and leave you both wide awake.

THAI MASSAGE

If your bathroom is big enough, and she's light enough, be ambitious and go for a Thai massage. This **soapy sex secret** from Southeast Asia is a great way to warm up for sex, or for cleaning yourselves afterwards. This full-body massage is usually given to a man by a woman, but with care he can return the favour. She lathers herself up with soapsuds while he lies on his front on a couple of towels on the floor. Once she's feeling foamy, she lies face down on his back and slips, slides and writhes up and down his body. He then turns over and she repeats the movements on his front. If he wants to return the favour, he should prop up his weight on his forearms like he does when he's on top during sex.

THERE'S THE RUB: APRÈS-SEX MASSAGE

Top athletes will also indulge in a massage after a big event to soothe aching muscles and prevent injury. Massaging your lover after sex extends your time together. These techniques can be used during foreplay, too, but many lovers say that massage after an orgasm is more relaxing as it can be enjoyed for its own sake, rather than as the prelude to intercourse – that is, unless you find that after using these sexy strokes on each other, you're ready for another bout of Sexercise!

Make sure the room is warm: even if you've worked up a sweat, it doesn't do for the muscles to become too cold as they can cramp up. If cranking up the central heating makes the

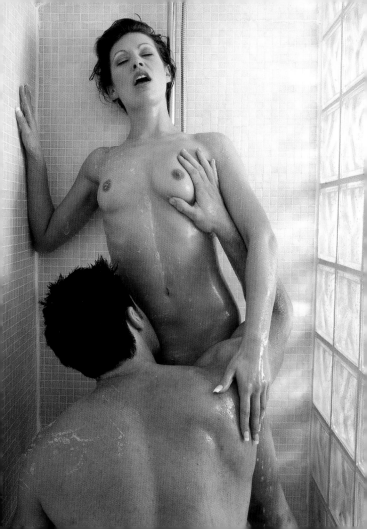

air seem too dry, place a bowl of water by the radiator to create some sexy humidity. Make sure you're both comfortable: many people like to place a towel on the floor, or use their bed, but a yoga mat covered in towels on the kitchen table means you can reach your partner without straining your back and the recipient of the massage has a comfortable place to lie.

Many masseurs use aromatherapy to help their clients wind down after a heavy workout and to enhance their mood and wellbeing. Essential oils from plants, herbs and flowers can be burned in an oil burner, or mixed in with plain massage oil (also available at chemists). Here are some you might like to try, depending on the mood you want to create.

Ylang-ylang is a powerful anti-depressant and is great if you want to talk while you're massaging each other as it enhances communication.

Lavender lowers stress levels and raises testosterone in men, so it's ideal if he's climaxed but she hasn't and would like to make love again.

Clary sage is a sedative: use this oil if you'd like to snuggle up and go to bed straight afterwards.

Basil will make you wide awake and clear your head: this is a great oil if you need to go out to work or for the evening after sex and is a good antidote for men who doze off after orgasm.

Rose is the ultimate special-occasion essential oil and especially loved by women because of its relaxing and luxurious qualities. Use it when you want to pamper her – pure rose oil is expensive, but great for anniversaries and birthdays.

Men love **sandalwood** as it's masculine and musky. Give him a sandalwood massage as a reward for a great sex session. It's also used to treat impotence, so a pre-sex massage using this oil is a good idea if he sometimes loses his erection.

SWISS TRICKS

Giving a massage can be intimidating the first time you try it, but if you concentrate on how your partner feels underneath your hands, you'll soon develop skills to rival any professional masseur. You'll learn to feel your way around your partner's body, to look for signs of tension and to listen for little clicks in the bones and muscles that show you where he or she is tense and stressed.

There are three basic techniques of Swiss massage, which was developed for *après-ski* muscle relaxing. Your hands should be clean, warm and free from jewellery. Warm the oil between your palms first, and keep replenishing it so your hands glide smoothly and continuously.

Effleurage: This technique uses long, gliding strokes to warm up your partner's muscles and to relax at the end. Use the whole of your hands flat on your partner's body with equal pressure coming down through the palms and the fingers. Contact should never be broken between your hands and your lover's body. Keep on moving, with at least one hand on your partner's body at all times. Used lightly, effleurage can tickle and tease; medium strokes will promote sleep; stronger ones will wake up and invigorate.

Petrissage: This is a more invigorating technique and involves kneading, squeezing and rolling fleshy areas of the body such as the stomach, thighs and buttocks. Take a portion of soft tissue between the thumb and the fingers on your hand and think of kneading dough: roll and squeeze the flesh between your hands, using your bodyweight to lean in and give weight to your strokes. It's fabulous for stiff or sprained muscles you've strained doing energetic positions as it gets the blood flowing to tender areas, soothing aches and pains.

Friction: Use the pads of your thumbs to make tiny circles on your partner's skin. You'll often need to use your bodyweight to provide the pressure required for this precise stroke. It's best for tight muscle spots, so necks, shoulders and thighs will benefit. It may not sound too sexy, but the more relaxed the muscles are, the more flexibility is improved, as is the ability to orgasm. So get making those circles!

AND FINALLY . . . THE GOLDEN RULE

Even if you can't create a spa environment to relax in, conclude your **Sexercise** experience by kissing each other, holding each other and talking about aspects of the experience you've enjoyed. That's the one unbreakable rule!

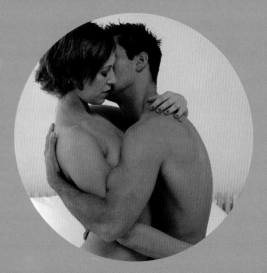